A COMPLETE 180
Tracking Your Weight Management Journey Over 180 Days

By

Innocent Karikoga

Balanced Life

Published by

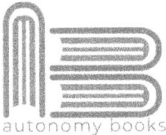

autonomy books

in collaboration with

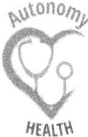

Autonomy

HEALTH

Balanced Life

No part of this publication may be reproduced, stored in a retrieval system, or transmitted in any form or by any means, electronic, mechanical, photocopying, and recording or otherwise, without the prior written permission of the author, except for brief passages in connection with a review written for publication or inclusion in a print or online medium, magazine, newspaper, periodical, or broadcast. To perform any of the aforementioned is an infringement of copyright law.

This publication provides content related to educational, medical, and psychological topics; however, it is not intended to be a substitute for the medical advice of a licensed physician. The reader should consult with their physician on any matters relating to his/her health. All matters regarding health require medical supervision. It is the responsibility of the reader to comply with their current and future medical treatments and advice. Further, understand that the guidance contained herein is not intended as a substitute for consultation with a licensed medical, educational, or health care professional, and usage of the material implies the acceptance of this disclaimer. Before beginning any change in lifestyle in any way, it is recommended to consult a licensed professional to ensure that you are doing what is best for your own health.

The intent of this book is to enlighten readers with a simplified and basic understanding of weight management and the way weight affects our bodies in a general sense.
The information found in this book is refined excerpts from the most recent editions of some of the most comprehensive medical textbooks. No claims without scientific explanations are found in this book.

First edition.

ISBN: 978-1-9994359-5-0

How To Use This Journal

This journal to track the progress of your weight management journey should be used complementary to **Balanced Life: Your Guide to Effective Weight Management.** You need to make **SMART** goals before you get started, that is, goals that are **Specific**, **Measurable**, **Achievable**, **Realistic**, and **Time-based**. For example, a 250lb woman may want to lose 50lbs in 6 months, which is specific, measurable, achievable, realistic, and time-based. However, while losing 100 lbs in 6 months for the same person might be specific, measurable, and time-based, that goal is likely not realistic and likely unachievable. Even if it could be achieved, it's not medically advisable to lose that much weight that quickly.

Before starting your weight loss journey, it's important to take some time to reflect and ask yourself the following fundamental questions:

1. Why do I want to lose weight? What are my specific health and/or personal goals?
2. What has stopped me from losing weight in the past, and how can I overcome those barriers?
3. Am I willing to make long-term lifestyle changes, rather than just pursuing a short-term "quick fix"?
4. How much weight do I realistically need to lose, and what is a safe and achievable rate of weight loss for me?

5. Do I have any underlying health conditions or physical limitations that might impact my weight loss journey?
6. What is my current diet, and how can I make sustainable changes to improve my eating habits?
7. What kind of exercise or physical activity do I enjoy, and how can I incorporate more of it into my weight loss routine?
8. How can I make sure I have a strong support system and accountability to keep me on track with my weight loss goals?
9. How will I measure my progress, and what will be my markers of success?
10. What are my potential triggers for overeating or bingeing, and how can I develop strategies to avoid or manage those triggers?

To help you in the next 180 days, you are highly advised to get a support network of either people who will go on this journey with you, or just be there for you as cheerleaders.

A Complete 180

Here are some fundamental tips for this 180-day weight loss journey that uses a mix of diet and exercise to encourage and achieve sustainable weight loss goals:

1. **Set Realistic Goals:** Before starting your weight loss journey, set realistic and achievable goals. For example, losing 1-2 pounds per week is a safe and sustainable rate of weight loss.

2. **Create a Meal Plan:** Create a healthy meal plan that includes a variety of whole, nutrient-dense foods such as fruits, vegetables, lean proteins, and whole grains. Limit processed and high-calorie foods.

3. **Track Your Food Intake:** Keeping track of what you eat can help you stay accountable and aware of your food choices.

4. **Exercise Regularly:** Start with moderate-intensity exercises such as walking, cycling or swimming, and gradually increase the intensity and frequency over time.

5. **Find Activities You Enjoy:** Choose exercises and physical activities that you enjoy, as it will make it easier to stick to your routine. This can be dancing, hiking, yoga, or team sports.

6. **Stay Hydrated:** Drink plenty of water, and avoid sugary drinks like soda and juice. Staying hydrated can help you avoid overeating, and it can also help boost your metabolism.

7. **Get Enough Sleep:** Aim for 7-8 hours of sleep per night. Getting enough sleep is essential for

weight loss because it helps you regulate hormones that control hunger and metabolism.

8. **Practice Mindful Eating:** Pay attention to your hunger and fullness cues. Learn to savour your food, eat slowly and mindfully, and avoid distractions like TV or phone while eating.

9. **Stay Motivated:** Keep yourself motivated by setting short-term and long-term goals, tracking your progress, and celebrating small victories along the way. Find a supportive community, or join a support group.

10. **Emphasize Sustainability:** Focus on creating healthy habits that you can maintain in the long term. Avoid fad diets or unsustainable exercise routines. Remember that weight loss is a journey, not a destination, and it requires consistent effort and patience.

A Complete 180

Common challenges to losing weight include:

- ❖ cravings and hunger
- ❖ emotional eating
- ❖ social pressures
- ❖ not enough time to prepare healthful foods
- ❖ lack of knowledge
- ❖ lack of motivation
- ❖ physical limitations
- ❖ lack of time to exercise
- ❖ access to resources

List your own challenges and how you plan to overcome them.

Challenge	Plan to overcome it
*Snacking on cake and ice-cream	*cut down on these gradually, while replacing them with apples and oranges

Balanced Life

List your goals that will serve as a guide to keep you on track. Remember to keep your goal S.M.A.R.T (Specific, Measurable, Achievable, Realistic, Time-based).

Short-term goals	Long-term goals
*To reduce caffeine intake on a defined weekly schedule.	*To completely stop consuming cafeine in 4 months

Balanced Life

A Complete 180

Example of how to fill out this journal

Meal	Food	Calories	Workout	Reps/ time	Sets
Breakfast	Fried Eggs, bread, orange juice	300, 300, 235	pushups Sit-ups Squats Plank	10 10 10 2 minutes	5 5 5 5
Snack	Apple, banana	50, 90	Full body stretches	--	--
Lunch	hamburger, fries, mango juice	300, 350, 235	pushups Sit-ups Squats Plank	10 10 10 2 minutes	5 5 5 5
Snack	Vegetable salad	100	Yoga	30 minutes	--
Dinner	Rice, chicken	200, 250	5km walk	60 minutes	--
Snack	Apple, banana	50, 90	Meditation	30 minutes	--
TCI*		2,550	DEE**	24*kg*1.5	TCI – DEE***

*Total Calorie Intake
** Daily Energy Expenditure = 24* weight (kg) * 1.5. Use 1.3 if you don't workout at all, and 1.7 if you're a professional athlete
*** TCI - DEE gives you your calorie deficit or calorie excess.
Notes
1. Aim for a 1% DEE difference from week to week. [DEE (week 1 day 1) – DEE (week 2 day 1)] / DEE (week 1 day 1) should be 1% or less.
2. PLEASE NOTE: It may take at least 6 weeks before you can consistently achieve the 1% reduction in DEE per week. For some, it may be easier to lose 1% of their weight in the few weeks before they plateau their DEE. In any case, it's essential to keep your focus on your ultimate goal and stay consistent with your diet and workout routine.
3. Feel free to take breaks, but you must complete at least 85% of the pages.
4. This journal should be used complementary to "Balanced Life: Your Comprehensive Guide to Effective Weight Management"

Balanced Life

"Your body is a reflection of your lifestyle. Make every choice a step toward a healthier, happier you."

Start date:

Week 1

Meal	Food	Calories	Workout	Reps	Sets
Breakfast					
Snack					
Lunch					
Snack					
Dinner					
Snack					
TCI			DEE		

A Complete 180

"Transform your body, transform your life. Every healthy choice is a step in the right direction."

Meal	Food	Calories	Workout	Reps	Sets
Breakfast					
Snack					
Lunch					
Snack					
Dinner					
Snack					
TCI			DEE		

Balanced Life

"Don't count the days; make the days count. Each workout, each meal choice is a victory on your journey."

Meal	Food	Calories	Workout	Reps	Sets
Breakfast					
Snack					
Lunch					
Snack					
Dinner					
Snack					
TCI			DEE		

A Complete 180

"Believe in the person you want to become. The journey may be tough, but the destination is worth it."

Meal	Food	Calories	Workout	Reps	Sets
Breakfast					
Snack					
Lunch					
Snack					
Dinner					
Snack					
TCI			DEE		

Balanced Life

"Progress, not perfection. Celebrate the small victories and keep pushing forward."

Meal	Food	Calories	Workout	Reps	Sets
Breakfast					
Snack					
Lunch					
Snack					
Dinner					
Snack					
TCI			DEE		

A Complete 180

"Your body is capable of amazing things. Fuel it with positivity, and watch the transformation unfold."

Meal	Food	Calories	Workout	Reps	Sets
Breakfast					
Snack					
Lunch					
Snack					
Dinner					
Snack					
TCI			DEE		

Balanced Life

"It's not about the weight you lose, but the life you gain. Embrace the journey, and let it empower you."

Meal	Food	Calories	Workout	Reps	Sets
Breakfast			LIGHT WORKOUT		
Snack			REST		
Lunch			LIGHT WORKOUT		
Snack			REST		
Dinner			LIGHT WORKOUT		
Snack			REST		
TCI			DEE		

A Complete 180

"Strive for progress, not perfection. Every step forward is a step toward a healthier, happier you."

Week 2

Meal	Food	Calories	Workout	Reps	Sets
Breakfast					
Snack					
Lunch					
Snack					
Dinner					
Snack					
TCI			DEE		

Balanced Life

"You have the power to sculpt the masterpiece that is your body. Take each workout as a stroke of the brush."

Meal	Food	Calories	Workout	Reps	Sets
Breakfast					
Snack					
Lunch					
Snack					
Dinner					
Snack					
TCI			DEE		

A Complete 180

"You are not on a diet; you are on a journey of self-discovery and self-love. Embrace the process, and let the results speak for themselves."

Meal	Food	Calories	Workout	Reps	Sets
Breakfast					
Snack					
Lunch					
Snack					
Dinner					
Snack					
TCI			DEE		

Balanced Life

"Your body hears everything your mind says. Speak words of strength, and watch your body follow suit."

Meal	Food	Calories	Workout	Reps	Sets
Breakfast					
Snack					
Lunch					
Snack					
Dinner					
Snack					
TCI			DEE		

A Complete 180

"Weight loss is not about the destination; it's about becoming the person who can achieve that goal."

Meal	Food	Calories	Workout	Reps	Sets
Breakfast					
Snack					
Lunch					
Snack					
Dinner					
Snack					
TCI			DEE		

Balanced Life

"The only bad workout is the one that didn't happen. Consistency is your strongest ally."

Meal	Food	Calories	Workout	Reps	Sets
Breakfast					
Snack					
Lunch					
Snack					
Dinner					
Snack					
TCI			DEE		

A Complete 180

"Sweat is magic; cover yourself in it daily to grant your body wishes of strength and transformation."

Meal	Food	Calories	Workout	Reps	Sets
Breakfast			LIGHT WORKOUT		
Snack			REST		
Lunch			LIGHT WORKOUT		
Snack			REST		
Dinner			LIGHT WORKOUT		
Snack			REST		
TCI			DEE		

Balanced Life

"Every workout is a step closer to your goals. Embrace the process, and trust the journey."

Week 3

Meal	Food	Calories	Workout	Reps	Sets
Breakfast					
Snack					
Lunch					
Snack					
Dinner					
Snack					
TCI			DEE		

A Complete 180

"Rise up, start fresh, and see the bright opportunity in each new day. Seize it!"

Meal	Food	Calories	Workout	Reps	Sets
Breakfast					
Snack					
Lunch					
Snack					
Dinner					
Snack					
TCI			DEE		

Balanced Life

"Your body is your home; treat it with love, nourishment, and the respect it deserves."

Meal	Food	Calories	Workout	Reps	Sets
Breakfast					
Snack					
Lunch					
Snack					
Dinner					
Snack					
TCI			DEE		

A Complete 180

"A journey of a thousand miles begins with a single step. Take that step today."

Meal	Food	Calories	Workout	Reps	Sets
Breakfast					
Snack					
Lunch					
Snack					
Dinner					
Snack					
TCI			DEE		

Balanced Life

"Fitness is not about being better than someone else; it's about being better than you used to be."

Meal	Food	Calories	Workout	Reps	Sets
Breakfast					
Snack					
Lunch					
Snack					
Dinner					
Snack					
TCI			DEE		

A Complete 180

"In the midst of challenges lies opportunity. Your weight loss journey is your canvas; paint it vibrant."

Meal	Food	Calories	Workout	Reps	Sets
Breakfast					
Snack					
Lunch					
Snack					
Dinner					
Snack					
TCI			DEE		

Balanced Life

"Believe you can, and you're halfway there. Trust the process, and the rest will follow."

Meal	Food	Calories	Workout	Reps	Sets
Breakfast			LIGHT WORKOUT		
Snack			REST		
Lunch			LIGHT WORKOUT		
Snack			REST		
Dinner			LIGHT WORKOUT		
Snack			REST		
TCI			DEE		

A Complete 180

"Fitness is not just about the body; it's a state of mind. Train your mind, and the body will follow."

Week 4

Meal	Food	Calories	Workout	Reps	Sets
Breakfast					
Snack					
Lunch					
Snack					
Dinner					
Snack					
TCI			DEE		

Balanced Life

"Every workout is a deposit into your health bank. Invest wisely, and the returns will amaze you."

Meal	Food	Calories	Workout	Reps	Sets
Breakfast					
Snack					
Lunch					
Snack					
Dinner					
Snack					
TCI			DEE		

A Complete 180

"Don't limit your challenges; challenge your limits. Break through barriers, and discover your strength."

Meal	Food	Calories	Workout	Reps	Sets
Breakfast					
Snack					
Lunch					
Snack					
Dinner					
Snack					
TCI			DEE		

Balanced Life
"You're not losing, you're gaining - gaining strength, confidence, and a healthier you."

Meal	Food	Calories	Workout	Reps	Sets
Breakfast					
Snack					
Lunch					
Snack					
Dinner					
Snack					
TCI			DEE		

A Complete 180

"The only thing standing between you and your goal is the story you keep telling yourself. Change the narrative."

Meal	Food	Calories	Workout	Reps	Sets
Breakfast					
Snack					
Lunch					
Snack					
Dinner					
Snack					
TCI			DEE		

Balanced Life

"Your journey is unique, just like you. Embrace the highs, learn from the lows, and keep moving forward."

Meal	Food	Calories	Workout	Reps	Sets
Breakfast					
Snack					
Lunch					
Snack					
Dinner					
Snack					
TCI			DEE		

A Complete 180

"You don't have to be great to start, but you have to start to be great. Begin your greatness today."

Meal	Food	Calories	Workout	Reps	Sets
Breakfast			LIGHT WORKOUT		
Snack			REST		
Lunch			LIGHT WORKOUT		
Snack			REST		
Dinner			LIGHT WORKOUT		
Snack			REST		
TCI			DEE		

Balanced Life

"Setbacks are setups for comebacks. Dust off, stand tall, and keep pushing forward."

Week 5

Meal	Food	Calories	Workout	Reps	Sets
Breakfast					
Snack					
Lunch					
Snack					
Dinner					
Snack					
TCI			DEE		

"Your body is an instrument, not an ornament. Play it well, and the symphony of health will follow."

Meal	Food	Calories	Workout	Reps	Sets
Breakfast					
Snack					
Lunch					
Snack					
Dinner					
Snack					
TCI			DEE		

Balanced Life

"Don't wait for inspiration; be the inspiration. Your journey might be someone else's motivation."

Meal	Food	Calories	Workout	Reps	Sets
Breakfast					
Snack					
Lunch					
Snack					
Dinner					
Snack					
TCI			DEE		

A Complete 180

"The only way to do great work is to love what you do. Fall in love with your journey."

Meal	Food	Calories	Workout	Reps	Sets
Breakfast					
Snack					
Lunch					
Snack					
Dinner					
Snack					
TCI			DEE		

Balanced Life

"Celebrate your progress, no matter how small. Each step forward is a victory worth acknowledging."

Meal	Food	Calories	Workout	Reps	Sets
Breakfast					
Snack					
Lunch					
Snack					
Dinner					
Snack					
TCI			DEE		

A Complete 180

"It's not about having time; it's about making time. Prioritize your health, and everything else will fall into place."

Meal	Food	Calories	Workout	Reps	Sets
Breakfast					
Snack					
Lunch					
Snack					
Dinner					
Snack					
TCI			DEE		

Balanced Life

"You are stronger than your excuses. Break free from limitations and embrace your potential."

Meal	Food	Calories	Workout	Reps	Sets
Breakfast			LIGHT WORKOUT		
Snack			REST		
Lunch			LIGHT WORKOUT		
Snack			REST		
Dinner			LIGHT WORKOUT		
Snack			REST		
TCI			DEE		

A Complete 180

**"The only bad workout is the one that didn't teach you something.
Every effort is a lesson in strength."**

Week 6

Meal	Food	Calories	Workout	Reps	Sets
Breakfast					
Snack					
Lunch					
Snack					
Dinner					
Snack					
TCI			DEE		

Balanced Life

"Transform fear into courage, doubts into determination, and obstacles into stepping stones."

Meal	Food	Calories	Workout	Reps	Sets
Breakfast					
Snack					
Lunch					
Snack					
Dinner					
Snack					
TCI			DEE		

A Complete 180

"Consistency is the key that unlocks the door to success. Keep turning that key every day."

Meal	Food	Calories	Workout	Reps	Sets
Breakfast					
Snack					
Lunch					
Snack					
Dinner					
Snack					
TCI			DEE		

Balanced Life

"Your body can withstand almost anything; it's your mind you need to convince. Believe, and you will achieve."

Meal	Food	Calories	Workout	Reps	Sets
Breakfast					
Snack					
Lunch					
Snack					
Dinner					
Snack					
TCI			DEE		

A Complete 180

"Your health is an investment, not an expense. Choose wisely, and watch your life flourish."

Meal	Food	Calories	Workout	Reps	Sets
Breakfast					
Snack					
Lunch					
Snack					
Dinner					
Snack					
TCI			DEE		

Balanced Life
"Success is not final, failure is not fatal: It's the courage to continue that counts. Keep going!"

Meal	Food	Calories	Workout	Reps	Sets
Breakfast					
Snack					
Lunch					
Snack					
Dinner					
Snack					
TCI			DEE		

A Complete 180

"A healthy outside starts from the inside. Nourish your body with love, and watch it thrive."

Meal	Food	Calories	Workout	Reps	Sets
Breakfast			LIGHT WORKOUT		
Snack			REST		
Lunch			LIGHT WORKOUT		
Snack			REST		
Dinner			LIGHT WORKOUT		
Snack			REST		
TCI			DEE		

Balanced Life
"Your body achieves what your mind believes. Feed it positivity, and let it conquer."

Week 7

Meal	Food	Calories	Workout	Reps	Sets
Breakfast					
Snack					
Lunch					
Snack					
Dinner					
Snack					
TCI			DEE		

A Complete 180

"Every step counts, every choice matters. You're not just losing weight; you're gaining a healthier, happier life."

Meal	Food	Calories	Workout	Reps	Sets
Breakfast					
Snack					
Lunch					
Snack					
Dinner					
Snack					
TCI			DEE		

Balanced Life

"Progress is progress, no matter how small. Celebrate each step forward on your journey."

Meal	Food	Calories	Workout	Reps	Sets
Breakfast					
Snack					
Lunch					
Snack					
Dinner					
Snack					
TCI			DEE		

A Complete 180

"Wake up with determination, go to bed with satisfaction. Repeat daily for a life-changing transformation."

Meal	Food	Calories	Workout	Reps	Sets
Breakfast					
Snack					
Lunch					
Snack					
Dinner					
Snack					
TCI			DEE		

Balanced Life

"Your journey is not defined by the scale but by the strength you discover along the way."

Meal	Food	Calories	Workout	Reps	Sets
Breakfast					
Snack					
Lunch					
Snack					
Dinner					
Snack					
TCI			DEE		

A Complete 180

**"Every day is a new opportunity to improve yourself. Seize it with
both hands and create a masterpiece."**

Meal	Food	Calories	Workout	Reps	Sets
Breakfast					
Snack					
Lunch					
Snack					
Dinner					
Snack					
TCI			DEE		

Balanced Life

"Your body is your most priceless possession; take care of it, nourish it, and it will reward you."

Meal	Food	Calories	Workout	Reps	Sets
Breakfast			LIGHT WORKOUT		
Snack			REST		
Lunch			LIGHT WORKOUT		
Snack			REST		
Dinner			LIGHT WORKOUT		
Snack			REST		
TCI			DEE		

A Complete 180

"Commit to your own success. Your journey is a reflection of the choices you make each day."

Week 8

Meal	Food	Calories	Workout	Reps	Sets
Breakfast					
Snack					
Lunch					
Snack					
Dinner					
Snack					
TCI			DEE		

Balanced Life

"Embrace the process, trust the journey, and remember: You are worth every drop of sweat, every healthy choice, and every step toward a better you."

Meal	Food	Calories	Workout	Reps	Sets
Breakfast					
Snack					
Lunch					
Snack					
Dinner					
Snack					
TCI			DEE		

A Complete 180

"Don't fear failure; fear being in the same place next year. Progress is the goal, perfection is the myth."

Meal	Food	Calories	Workout	Reps	Sets
Breakfast					
Snack					
Lunch					
Snack					
Dinner					
Snack					
TCI			DEE		

Balanced Life

"Health is not a destination; it's a lifelong journey. Enjoy the ride and savour each milestone."

Meal	Food	Calories	Workout	Reps	Sets
Breakfast					
Snack					
Lunch					
Snack					
Dinner					
Snack					
TCI			DEE		

A Complete 180

"The only limits that exist are the ones you place on yourself. Break free and soar to new heights."

Meal	Food	Calories	Workout	Reps	Sets
Breakfast					
Snack					
Lunch					
Snack					
Dinner					
Snack					
TCI			DEE		

Balanced Life

**"Small daily improvements are the key to long-term results.
Consistency compounds into significant change."**

Meal	Food	Calories	Workout	Reps	Sets
Breakfast					
Snack					
Lunch					
Snack					
Dinner					
Snack					
TCI			DEE		

A Complete 180

"Weight loss is not a sprint; it's a marathon. Pace yourself, stay focused, and cross that finish line with pride."

Meal	Food	Calories	Workout	Reps	Sets
Breakfast			LIGHT WORKOUT		
Snack			REST		
Lunch			LIGHT WORKOUT		
Snack			REST		
Dinner			LIGHT WORKOUT		
Snack			REST		
TCI			DEE		

Balanced Life

"Every decision matters. Choose progress over perfection, and let each positive choice propel you forward."

Week 9

Meal	Food	Calories	Workout	Reps	Sets
Breakfast					
Snack					
Lunch					
Snack					
Dinner					
Snack					
TCI			DEE		

A Complete 180

"Believe in your inner strength. You have the power to overcome any obstacle and transform your life."

Meal	Food	Calories	Workout	Reps	Sets
Breakfast					
Snack					
Lunch					
Snack					
Dinner					
Snack					
TCI			DEE		

Balanced Life

"Success is the sum of small efforts repeated daily. Keep pushing, keep striving, and success will follow."

Meal	Food	Calories	Workout	Reps	Sets
Breakfast					
Snack					
Lunch					
Snack					
Dinner					
Snack					
TCI			DEE		

A Complete 180

"Your body achieves what your mind believes. Visualize your success, and let that vision drive your journey."

Meal	Food	Calories	Workout	Reps	Sets
Breakfast					
Snack					
Lunch					
Snack					
Dinner					
Snack					
TCI			DEE		

Balanced Life

"Every day is a new opportunity to rewrite your story. Make it a story of strength, resilience, and triumph."

Meal	Food	Calories	Workout	Reps	Sets
Breakfast					
Snack					
Lunch					
Snack					
Dinner					
Snack					
TCI			DEE		

A Complete 180
"Your health is an investment, not an expense. The more you invest, the richer your life becomes."

Meal	Food	Calories	Workout	Reps	Sets
Breakfast					
Snack					
Lunch					
Snack					
Dinner					
Snack					
TCI			DEE		

Balanced Life
"Celebrate your non-scale victories. The way you feel and the energy you have are milestones, too."

Meal	Food	Calories	Workout	Reps	Sets
Breakfast			LIGHT WORKOUT		
Snack			REST		
Lunch			LIGHT WORKOUT		
Snack			REST		
Dinner			LIGHT WORKOUT		
Snack			REST		
TCI			DEE		

A Complete 180

"Be kind to yourself on this journey. Progress is progress, no matter the pace."

Week 10

Meal	Food	Calories	Workout	Reps	Sets
Breakfast					
Snack					
Lunch					
Snack					
Dinner					
Snack					
TCI			DEE		

Balanced Life

"Your body is your home; decorate it with health, fitness, and positivity."

Meal	Food	Calories	Workout	Reps	Sets
Breakfast					
Snack					
Lunch					
Snack					
Dinner					
Snack					
TCI			DEE		

A Complete 180

"Don't just lose weight; gain a lifestyle that radiates well-being and longevity."

Meal	Food	Calories	Workout	Reps	Sets
Breakfast					
Snack					
Lunch					
Snack					
Dinner					
Snack					
TCI			DEE		

Balanced Life

"You are the artist of your own health. Paint a vibrant picture with every choice you make."

Meal	Food	Calories	Workout	Reps	Sets
Breakfast					
Snack					
Lunch					
Snack					
Dinner					
Snack					
TCI			DEE		

A Complete 180

"Embrace the process of becoming the best version of yourself. It's a journey worth taking."

Meal	Food	Calories	Workout	Reps	Sets
Breakfast					
Snack					
Lunch					
Snack					
Dinner					
Snack					
TCI			DEE		

Balanced Life

"The road to success is paved with perseverance. Keep going; you're closer than you think."

Meal	Food	Calories	Workout	Reps	Sets
Breakfast					
Snack					
Lunch					
Snack					
Dinner					
Snack					
TCI			DEE		

A Complete 180

"Rome wasn't built in a day, nor is a healthy, resilient body. Patience is your greatest ally."

Meal	Food	Calories	Workout	Reps	Sets
Breakfast			LIGHT WORKOUT		
Snack			REST		
Lunch			LIGHT WORKOUT		
Snack			REST		
Dinner			LIGHT WORKOUT		
Snack			REST		
TCI			DEE		

Balanced Life
"Fitness is not a trend; it's a lifestyle. Embrace it, live it, and let it transform you."

Week 11

Meal	Food	Calories	Workout	Reps	Sets
Breakfast					
Snack					
Lunch					
Snack					
Dinner					
Snack					
TCI			DEE		

A Complete 180

"Your body is a reflection of your lifestyle choices. Choose wisely, and let your radiance shine through."

Meal	Food	Calories	Workout	Reps	Sets
Breakfast					
Snack					
Lunch					
Snack					
Dinner					
Snack					
TCI			DEE		

Balanced Life

"Create a vision that makes you want to jump out of bed in the morning. Let your fitness goals be that vision."

Meal	Food	Calories	Workout	Reps	Sets
Breakfast					
Snack					
Lunch					
Snack					
Dinner					
Snack					
TCI			DEE		

A Complete 180

"Transform your fear into fuel. Let it propel you toward a stronger, healthier you."

Meal	Food	Calories	Workout	Reps	Sets
Breakfast					
Snack					
Lunch					
Snack					
Dinner					
Snack					
TCI			DEE		

Balanced Life

"The journey may be tough, but remember: diamonds are made under pressure. Shine bright!"

Meal	Food	Calories	Workout	Reps	Sets
Breakfast					
Snack					
Lunch					
Snack					
Dinner					
Snack					
TCI			DEE		

A Complete 180

"Your body is capable of more than you think. Push beyond your limits, and discover your true strength."

Meal	Food	Calories	Workout	Reps	Sets
Breakfast					
Snack					
Lunch					
Snack					
Dinner					
Snack					
TCI			DEE		

Balanced Life

"Success is not just about the destination; it's about the person you become along the way."

Meal	Food	Calories	Workout	Reps	Sets
Breakfast			LIGHT WORKOUT		
Snack			REST		
Lunch			LIGHT WORKOUT		
Snack			REST		
Dinner			LIGHT WORKOUT		
Snack			REST		
TCI			DEE		

A Complete 180

"Make your health a priority, not an option. Your future self will thank you."

Week 12

Meal	Food	Calories	Workout	Reps	Sets
Breakfast					
Snack					
Lunch					
Snack					
Dinner					
Snack					
TCI			DEE		

Balanced Life

"Celebrate the milestones, no matter how small. Each step forward is a victory worth acknowledging."

Meal	Food	Calories	Workout	Reps	Sets
Breakfast					
Snack					
Lunch					
Snack					
Dinner					
Snack					
TCI			DEE		

A Complete 180

"Your journey is a testament to your strength and resilience. Keep going; you are writing your own success story."

Meal	Food	Calories	Workout	Reps	Sets
Breakfast					
Snack					
Lunch					
Snack					
Dinner					
Snack					
TCI			DEE		

Balanced Life
"Losing weight is not about restrictions; it's about gaining a life full of vitality and joy."

Meal	Food	Calories	Workout	Reps	Sets
Breakfast					
Snack					
Lunch					
Snack					
Dinner					
Snack					
TCI			DEE		

A Complete 180

"Fuel your body with self-love, nourishment, and determination. You are worth the effort."

Meal	Food	Calories	Workout	Reps	Sets
Breakfast					
Snack					
Lunch					
Snack					
Dinner					
Snack					
TCI			DEE		

Balanced Life

"Let go of the past; embrace the future. Your journey is about the person you are becoming."

Meal	Food	Calories	Workout	Reps	Sets
Breakfast					
Snack					
Lunch					
Snack					
Dinner					
Snack					
TCI			DEE		

A Complete 180

"You're not just shedding pounds; you're shedding self-doubt, limitations, and anything holding you back."

Meal	Food	Calories	Workout	Reps	Sets
Breakfast			LIGHT WORKOUT		
Snack			REST		
Lunch			LIGHT WORKOUT		
Snack			REST		
Dinner			LIGHT WORKOUT		
Snack			REST		
TCI			DEE		

Balanced Life

"See the beauty in the journey, not just the destination. Each step is a brushstroke on your canvas of success."

Week 13

Meal	Food	Calories	Workout	Reps	Sets
Breakfast					
Snack					
Lunch					
Snack					
Dinner					
Snack					
TCI			DEE		

A Complete 180

"Challenges are stepping stones, not roadblocks. Keep stepping, and watch your path unfold."

Meal	Food	Calories	Workout	Reps	Sets
Breakfast					
Snack					
Lunch					
Snack					
Dinner					
Snack					
TCI			DEE		

Balanced Life

"Your journey is a testament to your courage and resilience. Keep moving forward; you are stronger than you know."

Meal	Food	Calories	Workout	Reps	Sets
Breakfast					
Snack					
Lunch					
Snack					
Dinner					
Snack					
TCI			DEE		

A Complete 180

"You have the power to rewrite your story. Your journey is an evolution—embrace the transformation."

Meal	Food	Calories	Workout	Reps	Sets
Breakfast					
Snack					
Lunch					
Snack					
Dinner					
Snack					
TCI			DEE		

Balanced Life

"Every effort counts. Don't underestimate the power of consistent small steps toward your goals."

Meal	Food	Calories	Workout	Reps	Sets
Breakfast					
Snack					
Lunch					
Snack					
Dinner					
Snack					
TCI			DEE		

A Complete 180

"Your body is your home; treat it with love, respect, and the care it deserves. It's the only one you've got."

Meal	Food	Calories	Workout	Reps	Sets
Breakfast					
Snack					
Lunch					
Snack					
Dinner					
Snack					
TCI			DEE		

Balanced Life

"You're not just sculpting your body; you're crafting a life of vitality, strength, and endless possibilities."

Meal	Food	Calories	Workout	Reps	Sets
Breakfast			LIGHT WORKOUT		
Snack			REST		
Lunch			LIGHT WORKOUT		
Snack			REST		
Dinner			LIGHT WORKOUT		
Snack			REST		
TCI			DEE		

A Complete 180

"Turn your 'I can't' into 'I will.' The first step to success is believing in your own potential."

Week 14

Meal	Food	Calories	Workout	Reps	Sets
Breakfast					
Snack					
Lunch					
Snack					
Dinner					
Snack					
TCI			DEE		

Balanced Life

"Fitness is not just a physical journey; it's a mental and emotional transformation. Embrace the whole process."

Meal	Food	Calories	Workout	Reps	Sets
Breakfast					
Snack					
Lunch					
Snack					
Dinner					
Snack					
TCI			DEE		

A Complete 180

"Your journey is not a sprint; it's a marathon of self-discovery and personal triumphs."

Meal	Food	Calories	Workout	Reps	Sets
Breakfast					
Snack					
Lunch					
Snack					
Dinner					
Snack					
TCI			DEE		

Balanced Life

"Invest in your health today; it's the greatest gift you can give your future self."

Meal	Food	Calories	Workout	Reps	Sets
Breakfast					
Snack					
Lunch					
Snack					
Dinner					
Snack					
TCI			DEE		

A Complete 180

"Find joy in the journey. The more you enjoy the process, the more sustainable your progress becomes."

Meal	Food	Calories	Workout	Reps	Sets
Breakfast					
Snack					
Lunch					
Snack					
Dinner					
Snack					
TCI			DEE		

Balanced Life

"You're not just shedding weight; you're gaining a renewed sense of confidence and self-worth."

Meal	Food	Calories	Workout	Reps	Sets
Breakfast					
Snack					
Lunch					
Snack					
Dinner					
Snack					
TCI			DEE		

A Complete 180

"Every sweat session is a love letter to your body. Cherish the effort; it's a celebration of self-care."

Meal	Food	Calories	Workout	Reps	Sets
Breakfast			LIGHT WORKOUT		
Snack			REST		
Lunch			LIGHT WORKOUT		
Snack			REST		
Dinner			LIGHT WORKOUT		
Snack			REST		
TCI			DEE		

Balanced Life

"In the dance of progress, every step counts. Keep dancing, and watch the rhythm of your success unfold."

Week 15

Meal	Food	Calories	Workout	Reps	Sets
Breakfast					
Snack					
Lunch					
Snack					
Dinner					
Snack					
TCI			DEE		

A Complete 180

"Remember, it's not about the destination; it's about who you become on the way there. Keep evolving, keep growing."

Meal	Food	Calories	Workout	Reps	Sets
Breakfast					
Snack					
Lunch					
Snack					
Dinner					
Snack					
TCI			DEE		

Balanced Life

"Your journey is a symphony of strength. Every workout, every healthy meal, contributes to the beautiful melody of your success."

Meal	Food	Calories	Workout	Reps	Sets
Breakfast					
Snack					
Lunch					
Snack					
Dinner					
Snack					
TCI			DEE		

A Complete 180

"The journey may be challenging, but you're forging resilience with every step. You're not just losing weight; you're gaining strength."

Meal	Food	Calories	Workout	Reps	Sets
Breakfast					
Snack					
Lunch					
Snack					
Dinner					
Snack					
TCI			DEE		

Balanced Life

"Your body is your masterpiece in the making. Sculpt it with determination, paint it with positivity, and admire the work of art you become."

Meal	Food	Calories	Workout	Reps	Sets
Breakfast					
Snack					
Lunch					
Snack					
Dinner					
Snack					
TCI			DEE		

"Don't just break a sweat; break through barriers. Every challenge is an opportunity to discover your untapped potential."

Meal	Food	Calories	Workout	Reps	Sets
Breakfast					
Snack					
Lunch					
Snack					
Dinner					
Snack					
TCI			DEE		

Balanced Life

"Your journey is a testament to your commitment. Keep pushing, keep striving; the transformation is happening with every effort."

Meal	Food	Calories	Workout	Reps	Sets
Breakfast			LIGHT WORKOUT		
Snack			REST		
Lunch			LIGHT WORKOUT		
Snack			REST		
Dinner			LIGHT WORKOUT		
Snack			REST		
TCI			DEE		

A Complete 180

**"Health is not a destination you reach; it's a way of life you
cultivate. Enjoy the journey, and let it unfold naturally."**

Week 16

Meal	Food	Calories	Workout	Reps	Sets
Breakfast					
Snack					
Lunch					
Snack					
Dinner					
Snack					
TCI			DEE		

Balanced Life

"You're rewriting your story with every healthy choice. Let each chapter be a celebration of your strength and resilience."

Meal	Food	Calories	Workout	Reps	Sets
Breakfast					
Snack					
Lunch					
Snack					
Dinner					
Snack					
TCI			DEE		

A Complete 180

"Celebrate the process, not just the progress. The journey is where you discover your true capabilities."

Meal	Food	Calories	Workout	Reps	Sets
Breakfast					
Snack					
Lunch					
Snack					
Dinner					
Snack					
TCI			DEE		

Balanced Life

"Your body hears the whispers of self-love. Speak kindly to yourself, and watch how your body responds with strength and vitality."

Meal	Food	Calories	Workout	Reps	Sets
Breakfast					
Snack					
Lunch					
Snack					
Dinner					
Snack					
TCI			DEE		

A Complete 180

"Every challenge is an opportunity in disguise. Embrace the difficulties; they are stepping stones on your path to success."

Meal	Food	Calories	Workout	Reps	Sets
Breakfast					
Snack					
Lunch					
Snack					
Dinner					
Snack					
TCI			DEE		

Balanced Life
"Success is not found in the destination; it's found in the daily disciplines that lead you there. Be disciplined, be successful."

Meal	Food	Calories	Workout	Reps	Sets
Breakfast					
Snack					
Lunch					
Snack					
Dinner					
Snack					
TCI			DEE		

"Your health is an investment, not an expense. The dividends include vitality, joy, and a life well-lived."

Meal	Food	Calories	Workout	Reps	Sets
Breakfast			LIGHT WORKOUT		
Snack			REST		
Lunch			LIGHT WORKOUT		
Snack			REST		
Dinner			LIGHT WORKOUT		
Snack			REST		
TCI			DEE		

Balanced Life

"It's not about perfection; it's about progress. Keep moving forward, and celebrate the progress you make along the way."

Week 17

Meal	Food	Calories	Workout	Reps	Sets
Breakfast					
Snack					
Lunch					
Snack					
Dinner					
Snack					
TCI			DEE		

A Complete 180

"Fitness is not just about the body; it's about the mindset. Train your mind, and your body will follow."

Meal	Food	Calories	Workout	Reps	Sets
Breakfast					
Snack					
Lunch					
Snack					
Dinner					
Snack					
TCI			DEE		

Balanced Life

"Your journey is a mosaic of dedication and resilience. Each piece, no matter how small, contributes to the beautiful picture of your success."

Meal	Food	Calories	Workout	Reps	Sets
Breakfast					
Snack					
Lunch					
Snack					
Dinner					
Snack					
TCI			DEE		

A Complete 180

"In the dance of transformation, every move counts. Dance to the rhythm of your heartbeat and feel the energy of your success."

Meal	Food	Calories	Workout	Reps	Sets
Breakfast					
Snack					
Lunch					
Snack					
Dinner					
Snack					
TCI			DEE		

Balanced Life
"Your body is a canvas; sculpt it with purpose, paint it with positivity, and create a masterpiece that reflects your strength."

Meal	Food	Calories	Workout	Reps	Sets
Breakfast					
Snack					
Lunch					
Snack					
Dinner					
Snack					
TCI			DEE		

A Complete 180

"The journey may be tough, but so are you. Every challenge is an opportunity for growth and a step closer to your goals."

Meal	Food	Calories	Workout	Reps	Sets
Breakfast					
Snack					
Lunch					
Snack					
Dinner					
Snack					
TCI			DEE		

Balanced Life

"The journey is not about finding yourself; it's about creating yourself. You're sculpting a stronger, more vibrant you with every healthy choice."

Meal	Food	Calories	Workout	Reps	Sets
Breakfast			LIGHT WORKOUT		
Snack			REST		
Lunch			LIGHT WORKOUT		
Snack			REST		
Dinner			LIGHT WORKOUT		
Snack			REST		
TCI			DEE		

A Complete 180

"Your strength is your superpower. Channel it, embrace it, and let it guide you to a healthier, happier you."

Week 18

Meal	Food	Calories	Workout	Reps	Sets
Breakfast					
Snack					
Lunch					
Snack					
Dinner					
Snack					
TCI			DEE		

Balanced Life

"Your journey is a story of triumph over challenges. Keep writing, keep rewriting, and let the narrative be one of strength and resilience."

Meal	Food	Calories	Workout	Reps	Sets
Breakfast					
Snack					
Lunch					
Snack					
Dinner					
Snack					
TCI			DEE		

A Complete 180

"Every healthy choice is a love note to your body. Shower it affectionately, and watch it respond with vitality and strength."

Meal	Food	Calories	Workout	Reps	Sets
Breakfast					
Snack					
Lunch					
Snack					
Dinner					
Snack					
TCI			DEE		

Balanced Life

**"The journey may be uphill, but the view from the top is worth it.
Keep climbing; your summit is within reach."**

Meal	Food	Calories	Workout	Reps	Sets
Breakfast					
Snack					
Lunch					
Snack					
Dinner					
Snack					
TCI			DEE		

A Complete 180

"Your body is your ally, not your enemy. Treat it with kindness, and it will reward you with resilience and well-being."

Meal	Food	Calories	Workout	Reps	Sets
Breakfast					
Snack					
Lunch					
Snack					
Dinner					
Snack					
TCI			DEE		

Balanced Life

"Life is a journey, and so is your health. Embrace the twists, turns, and detours, knowing each step is part of your unique path."

Meal	Food	Calories	Workout	Reps	Sets
Breakfast					
Snack					
Lunch					
Snack					
Dinner					
Snack					
TCI			DEE		

A Complete 180

"Progress is not always visible on the outside; it's often felt on the inside. Feel the strength growing within you with every effort."

Meal	Food	Calories	Workout	Reps	Sets
Breakfast			LIGHT WORKOUT		
Snack			REST		
Lunch			LIGHT WORKOUT		
Snack			REST		
Dinner			LIGHT WORKOUT		
Snack			REST		
TCI			DEE		

Balanced Life
"Your health is your wealth. Invest in it daily, and watch the abundance of well-being unfold in your life."

Week 19

Meal	Food	Calories	Workout	Reps	Sets
Breakfast					
Snack					
Lunch					
Snack					
Dinner					
Snack					
TCI			DEE		

A Complete 180

"Every bead of sweat is a testament to your dedication. Let it glisten as a badge of honour on your journey."

Meal	Food	Calories	Workout	Reps	Sets
Breakfast					
Snack					
Lunch					
Snack					
Dinner					
Snack					
TCI			DEE		

Balanced Life

"Transform the 'I can't' into 'I am.' Affirm your strength, and watch how your body responds to the power of self-belief."

Meal	Food	Calories	Workout	Reps	Sets
Breakfast					
Snack					
Lunch					
Snack					
Dinner					
Snack					
TCI			DEE		

A Complete 180

"Your journey is a mosaic of choices. Piece by piece, decision by decision, you're creating a masterpiece of health and vitality."

Meal	Food	Calories	Workout	Reps	Sets
Breakfast					
Snack					
Lunch					
Snack					
Dinner					
Snack					
TCI			DEE		

Balanced Life

"Your body is a temple. Treat it with reverence, nourish it with care, and let it radiate with the glow of well-being."

Meal	Food	Calories	Workout	Reps	Sets
Breakfast					
Snack					
Lunch					
Snack					
Dinner					
Snack					
TCI			DEE		

A Complete 180

"Celebrate the progress, no matter how small. Each step forward is a victory on your journey to a healthier you."

Meal	Food	Calories	Workout	Reps	Sets
Breakfast					
Snack					
Lunch					
Snack					
Dinner					
Snack					
TCI			DEE		

Balanced Life

"You're not just losing weight; you're gaining strength, confidence, and a profound connection with your own resilience."

Meal	Food	Calories	Workout	Reps	Sets
Breakfast			LIGHT WORKOUT		
Snack			REST		
Lunch			LIGHT WORKOUT		
Snack			REST		
Dinner			LIGHT WORKOUT		
Snack			REST		
TCI			DEE		

A Complete 180

"Every challenge you overcome is a milestone in your journey. Embrace them; they're leading you to your best self."

Week 20

Meal	Food	Calories	Workout	Reps	Sets
Breakfast					
Snack					
Lunch					
Snack					
Dinner					
Snack					
TCI			DEE		

Balanced Life

"Your journey is a testament to your commitment to self-improvement. Keep going, keep growing, and let each day be a step forward."

Meal	Food	Calories	Workout	Reps	Sets
Breakfast					
Snack					
Lunch					
Snack					
Dinner					
Snack					
TCI			DEE		

A Complete 180

"Strive for progress, not perfection. Your journey is about improvement, not unrealistic standards."

Meal	Food	Calories	Workout	Reps	Sets
Breakfast					
Snack					
Lunch					
Snack					
Dinner					
Snack					
TCI			DEE		

Balanced Life

"Your health journey is a marathon, not a sprint. Pace yourself, stay focused, and celebrate the endurance you're building."

Meal	Food	Calories	Workout	Reps	Sets
Breakfast					
Snack					
Lunch					
Snack					
Dinner					
Snack					
TCI			DEE		

A Complete 180

"See each healthy choice as a seed planted. Nurture them, and watch your health and well-being bloom."

Meal	Food	Calories	Workout	Reps	Sets
Breakfast					
Snack					
Lunch					
Snack					
Dinner					
Snack					
TCI			DEE		

Balanced Life

"Your body is an instrument; play it with care, love, and the beautiful music of a healthy, active lifestyle."

Meal	Food	Calories	Workout	Reps	Sets
Breakfast					
Snack					
Lunch					
Snack					
Dinner					
Snack					
TCI			DEE		

A Complete 180

"Every step forward is a leap toward a healthier, happier you. Your journey is a series of these powerful leaps."

Meal	Food	Calories	Workout	Reps	Sets
Breakfast			LIGHT WORKOUT		
Snack			REST		
Lunch			LIGHT WORKOUT		
Snack			REST		
Dinner			LIGHT WORKOUT		
Snack			REST		
TCI			DEE		

Balanced Life

"In the gallery of your life, let your health journey be the masterpiece that captures attention, admiration, and inspiration."

Week 21

Meal	Food	Calories	Workout	Reps	Sets
Breakfast					
Snack					
Lunch					
Snack					
Dinner					
Snack					
TCI			DEE		

A Complete 180

"Every day is a new chapter in your health journey. Write it with purpose, dedication, and the ink of positive choices."

Meal	Food	Calories	Workout	Reps	Sets
Breakfast					
Snack					
Lunch					
Snack					
Dinner					
Snack					
TCI			DEE		

Balanced Life

"Your journey is a personal revolution. Revolt against self-doubt, unhealthy habits, and limitations. You are the architect of your transformation."

Meal	Food	Calories	Workout	Reps	Sets
Breakfast					
Snack					
Lunch					
Snack					
Dinner					
Snack					
TCI			DEE		

A Complete 180

"The journey may have challenges, but each challenge is a teacher, guiding you toward greater strength and resilience."

Meal	Food	Calories	Workout	Reps	Sets
Breakfast					
Snack					
Lunch					
Snack					
Dinner					
Snack					
TCI			DEE		

Balanced Life

"Your body is a work in progress, and so is your journey. Embrace both with patience, dedication, and a commitment to growth."

Meal	Food	Calories	Workout	Reps	Sets
Breakfast					
Snack					
Lunch					
Snack					
Dinner					
Snack					
TCI			DEE		

A Complete 180

"Celebrate the process, not just the outcome. The journey is where you discover your inner strength and capacity for growth."

Meal	Food	Calories	Workout	Reps	Sets
Breakfast					
Snack					
Lunch					
Snack					
Dinner					
Snack					
TCI			DEE		

Balanced Life

"Every healthy choice is a vote for a vibrant, energetic life. Choose wisely, and watch your health flourish."

Meal	Food	Calories	Workout	Reps	Sets
Breakfast			LIGHT WORKOUT		
Snack			REST		
Lunch			LIGHT WORKOUT		
Snack			REST		
Dinner			LIGHT WORKOUT		
Snack			REST		
TCI			DEE		

A Complete 180

"Your journey is an unfolding story of courage, strength, and resilience. Keep writing the chapters that lead to a healthier you."

Week 22

Meal	Food	Calories	Workout	Reps	Sets
Breakfast					
Snack					
Lunch					
Snack					
Dinner					
Snack					
TCI			DEE		

Balanced Life

"Your health is an investment in your future. Plant the seeds today for a life of abundance in well-being."

Meal	Food	Calories	Workout	Reps	Sets
Breakfast					
Snack					
Lunch					
Snack					
Dinner					
Snack					
TCI			DEE		

A Complete 180

"Your journey is not just about physical transformation; it's about evolving into the best version of yourself. Embrace the evolution."

Meal	Food	Calories	Workout	Reps	Sets
Breakfast					
Snack					
Lunch					
Snack					
Dinner					
Snack					
TCI			DEE		

Balanced Life

"Celebrate the process, not just the progress. The journey is where you discover your strength and resilience."

Meal	Food	Calories	Workout	Reps	Sets
Breakfast					
Snack					
Lunch					
Snack					
Dinner					
Snack					
TCI			DEE		

A Complete 180

"In every challenge, there's an opportunity to grow. Embrace the challenges; they're stepping stones to your success."

Meal	Food	Calories	Workout	Reps	Sets
Breakfast					
Snack					
Lunch					
Snack					
Dinner					
Snack					
TCI			DEE		

Balanced Life

"Your health journey is a gift to your future self. Unwrap it with dedication, love, and a commitment to lasting well-being."

Meal	Food	Calories	Workout	Reps	Sets
Breakfast					
Snack					
Lunch					
Snack					
Dinner					
Snack					
TCI			DEE		

A Complete 180

"See every workout as an investment in yourself. The dividends are not just physical; they're mental and emotional too."

Meal	Food	Calories	Workout	Reps	Sets
Breakfast			LIGHT WORKOUT		
Snack			REST		
Lunch			LIGHT WORKOUT		
Snack			REST		
Dinner			LIGHT WORKOUT		
Snack			REST		
TCI			DEE		

Balanced Life

**"Transform the desire for change into the commitment to change.
Your dedication is the catalyst for a healthier, happier you."**

Week 23

Meal	Food	Calories	Workout	Reps	Sets
Breakfast					
Snack					
Lunch					
Snack					
Dinner					
Snack					
TCI			DEE		

A Complete 180

**"Every drop of sweat is a testament to your effort and dedication.
Let it be the ink that writes your story of triumph."**

Meal	Food	Calories	Workout	Reps	Sets
Breakfast					
Snack					
Lunch					
Snack					
Dinner					
Snack					
TCI			DEE		

Balanced Life

"Your journey is an opportunity to rediscover your strength. With every challenge, you're unveiling the power within."

Meal	Food	Calories	Workout	Reps	Sets
Breakfast					
Snack					
Lunch					
Snack					
Dinner					
Snack					
TCI			DEE		

A Complete 180

"Your health is your wealth, and every positive choice is a deposit into your well-being bank. Invest wisely."

Meal	Food	Calories	Workout	Reps	Sets
Breakfast					
Snack					
Lunch					
Snack					
Dinner					
Snack					
TCI			DEE		

Balanced Life

"Celebrate the victories, no matter how small. Each one is a sign of progress on your transformative journey."

Meal	Food	Calories	Workout	Reps	Sets
Breakfast					
Snack					
Lunch					
Snack					
Dinner					
Snack					
TCI			DEE		

A Complete 180
"The journey to health is not a race; it's a conscious, deliberate, and sustainable march toward a better version of yourself."

Meal	Food	Calories	Workout	Reps	Sets
Breakfast					
Snack					
Lunch					
Snack					
Dinner					
Snack					
TCI			DEE		

Balanced Life

"Your body is your ally in this journey. Treat it with kindness, fuel it with nourishment, and watch it respond with vitality."

Meal	Food	Calories	Workout	Reps	Sets
Breakfast			LIGHT WORKOUT		
Snack			REST		
Lunch			LIGHT WORKOUT		
Snack			REST		
Dinner			LIGHT WORKOUT		
Snack			REST		
TCI			DEE		

A Complete 180

"The journey may have ups and downs, but every twist and turn is crafting a story of resilience and determination."

Week 24

Meal	Food	Calories	Workout	Reps	Sets
Breakfast					
Snack					
Lunch					
Snack					
Dinner					
Snack					
TCI			DEE		

"See every obstacle as a challenge to overcome, not a barrier to your progress. Your journey is about conquering."

Meal	Food	Calories	Workout	Reps	Sets
Breakfast					
Snack					
Lunch					
Snack					
Dinner					
Snack					
TCI			DEE		

"The journey is not just about losing weight; it's about gaining confidence, self-love, and a profound sense of well-being."

Meal	Food	Calories	Workout	Reps	Sets
Breakfast					
Snack					
Lunch					
Snack					
Dinner					
Snack					
TCI			DEE		

Balanced Life

"Celebrate the journey, for it's where you discover the strength you didn't know you had and the person you're becoming."

Meal	Food	Calories	Workout	Reps	Sets
Breakfast					
Snack					
Lunch					
Snack					
Dinner					
Snack					
TCI			DEE		

"In the tapestry of your life, let your health journey be the vibrant thread that weaves a story of strength and triumph."

Meal	Food	Calories	Workout	Reps	Sets
Breakfast					
Snack					
Lunch					
Snack					
Dinner					
Snack					
TCI			DEE		

Balanced Life

"In the narrative of your life, let your health journey be the chapter that highlights your strength, resilience, and unwavering dedication."

Meal	Food	Calories	Workout	Reps	Sets
Breakfast					
Snack					
Lunch					
Snack					
Dinner					
Snack					
TCI			DEE		

"Your journey is an evolution. Each step forward is a metamorphosis into a healthier, more empowered version of yourself."

Meal	Food	Calories	Workout	Reps	Sets
Breakfast			LIGHT WORKOUT		
Snack			REST		
Lunch			LIGHT WORKOUT		
Snack			REST		
Dinner			LIGHT WORKOUT		
Snack			REST		
TCI			DEE		

Balanced Life

"Celebrate the milestones, but also cherish the daily efforts. Your journey is a mosaic of consistent dedication."

Week 25

Meal	Food	Calories	Workout	Reps	Sets
Breakfast					
Snack					
Lunch					
Snack					
Dinner					
Snack					
TCI			DEE		

A Complete 180

"Your health journey is not just about physical change; it's a holistic transformation that encompasses mind, body, and spirit."

Meal	Food	Calories	Workout	Reps	Sets
Breakfast					
Snack					
Lunch					
Snack					
Dinner					
Snack					
TCI			DEE		

Balanced Life

"Each healthy choice is a brushstroke painting on the canvas of your health journey. Create a masterpiece."

Meal	Food	Calories	Workout	Reps	Sets
Breakfast					
Snack					
Lunch					
Snack					
Dinner					
Snack					
TCI			DEE		

A Complete 180

"The journey may be challenging, but remember: diamonds are formed under pressure. Shine bright on your path to success."

Meal	Food	Calories	Workout	Reps	Sets
Breakfast					
Snack					
Lunch					
Snack					
Dinner					
Snack					
TCI			DEE		

Balanced Life

"Your body is the sculpture, and each workout is a chisel shaping it into a masterpiece of strength and vitality."

Meal	Food	Calories	Workout	Reps	Sets
Breakfast					
Snack					
Lunch					
Snack					
Dinner					
Snack					
TCI			DEE		

"In the orchestra of your life, let your health journey be the melody that resonates with energy, positivity, and well-being."

Meal	Food	Calories	Workout	Reps	Sets
Breakfast					
Snack					
Lunch					
Snack					
Dinner					
Snack					
TCI			DEE		

Balanced Life

"See every challenge as a stepping stone. Your journey is about rising above obstacles and reaching new heights."

Meal	Food	Calories	Workout	Reps	Sets
Breakfast			LIGHT WORKOUT		
Snack			REST		
Lunch			LIGHT WORKOUT		
Snack			REST		
Dinner			LIGHT WORKOUT		
Snack			REST		
TCI			DEE		

A Complete 180

"Celebrate not just the physical changes, but also the mental and emotional strength you're gaining on your journey."

Week 26

Meal	Food	Calories	Workout	Reps	Sets
Breakfast					
Snack					
Lunch					
Snack					
Dinner					
Snack					
TCI			DEE		

Balanced Life

"Your journey is a dance of determination. Move to the rhythm of your goals and let every step express your commitment."

Meal	Food	Calories	Workout	Reps	Sets
Breakfast					
Snack					
Lunch					
Snack					
Dinner					
Snack					
TCI			DEE		

A Complete 180

"Your health journey is a marathon, not a sprint. Pace yourself, stay committed, and savour the endurance you're building."

Meal	Food	Calories	Workout	Reps	Sets
Breakfast					
Snack					
Lunch					
Snack					
Dinner					
Snack					
TCI			DEE		

Balanced Life

"See every setback as a setup for a comeback. Your journey is a series of comebacks that make you stronger."

Meal	Food	Calories	Workout	Reps	Sets
Breakfast					
Snack					
Lunch					
Snack					
Dinner					
Snack					
TCI			DEE		

A Complete 180

**"Every positive choice is a step toward a brighter, healthier future.
Your journey is a testament to your commitment."**

Meal	Food	Calories	Workout	Reps	Sets
Breakfast					
Snack					
Lunch					
Snack					
Dinner					
Snack					
TCI			DEE		

Balanced Life

"Celebrate your journey as a testament to your courage and commitment. You're not just transforming your body; you're transforming your life."

Meal	Food	Calories	Workout	Reps	Sets
Breakfast					
Snack					
Lunch					
Snack					
Dinner					
Snack					
TCI			DEE		

A Complete 180

"Every moment of discomfort is a step closer to your goal. Embrace the challenge, for it's shaping a stronger, resilient you."

Meal	Food	Calories	Workout	Reps	Sets
Breakfast			LIGHT WORKOUT		
Snack			REST		
Lunch			LIGHT WORKOUT		
Snack			REST		
Dinner			LIGHT WORKOUT		
Snack			REST		
TCI			DEE		

Congratulations!

A Complete 180

Feel like you're on a roll and want to keep going?

First, take a break for a week, then get back to it.

Remind yourself that you're awesome every step of the way.

www.ingramcontent.com/pod-product-compliance
Lightning Source LLC
Chambersburg PA
CBHW062134020426
42335CB00013B/1216